T0023081

PAJAMA
PILATES

PAJAMA PILATES

40 EXERCISES
for Stretching, Strengthening, and Toning at Home

MARIA MANKIN

Illustrations by **MAJA TOMLJANOVIC**

CHRONICLE BOOKS
SAN FRANCISCO

Text copyright © 2021 by Maria Mankin.

All rights reserved. No part of this book
may be reproduced in any form without
written permission from the publisher.

Library of Congress Cataloging-in-Publication Data
available.

ISBN: 978-1-7972-0708-7

Manufactured in China.

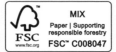

Artwork by Maja Tomljanovic.
Design by Lizzie Vaughan.
Typeset in Swiss 721.

The information contained in *Pajama Pilates* is
presented for educational purposes only. This book
is in no way intended as a substitute for the medical
advice of physicians. If you seek to treat a physical
condition using Pilates practices, please consult with
your physician or a licensed healthcare provider first.

10 9 8 7 6 5 4

Chronicle books and gifts are available at special
quantity discounts to corporations, professional
associations, literacy programs, and other
organizations. For details and discount information,
please contact our premiums department at
corporatesales@chroniclebooks.com or at
1-800-759-0190.

Chronicle Books LLC
680 Second Street
San Francisco, California 94107
www.chroniclebooks.com

TO LINA,

my mother, whose creativity,
strength, and love have
empowered and inspired me
throughout the years.

CONTENTS

PILATES IN YOUR PAJAMAS

Welcome to Pajama Pilates (or Pajamalates, as I like to call it),
an at-home Pilates practice—that's right, you've guessed it—
done in your pajamas!

Whether in your bedroom, kitchen, bathroom, or living room, you can do the forty Pilates exercises included in this book without leaving your house, or even getting dressed. Based on the world-renowned exercise system developed 100 years ago by Joseph Pilates, Pajama Pilates is a well-rounded strengthening, stretching, and toning program for every age and skill level. It targets all major areas of your body, helping you become fit, strong, and healthy by improving flexibility, core strength, posture, and coordination, and also fosters a holistic sense of vitality, well-being, and balance.

THE PROGRAM

One of the most important parts of any Pilates program is committing to a consistent practice. With Pajama Pilates, you can exercise in the comfort of your own home, turning your house into a private gym, and avoid schlepping to and from fitness classes across town. This book provides simple exercises to be done in different areas of your house, using furniture—like your bed, sofa, and bathtub—as props. No fancy equipment is necessary. All that's needed to have fun and get fit with Pajama Pilates are common household items—like a pillow and a couple of soup cans.

ABOUT ME AND MY INSPIRATION

In my twenties, I moved from Sicily to San Francisco to run away with a small one-ring circus. Our circus had no lion tamers or chimpanzees riding unicycles, but I performed daring acrobatic routines that were hard on my body. If I could, today, I would whisper in the ear of my younger self: "Hey, be smart: Do Pilates!" In fact, a good regimen like Pajama Pilates would have served me well during my career as an acrobat.

A few years after joining the circus, I stumbled into Pilates after falling from my husband's shoulders doing a difficult stunt, the "Jump Rope of Death," in Yosemite National Park—yes, a tad unusual but, for me, just a day at the office. I injured my back and tore ligaments along my right elbow. After only a couple of Pilates sessions, I started to feel stronger and more aware of my body. My injuries slowly healed, and I fell in love with the practice. Pilates changed my body even beyond my initial recovery, but my true aha moment happened when I realized my love of sharing Pilates with other people. So, I became an instructor. For years, I jotted down and sketched out exercises for my clients so they could do them at home. One day, a favorite work-from-home client asked for a list of exercises to do in bed in the morning, so I drew her doing them in her pajamas. We started calling it Pajamalates; eventually it just stuck. And, of course, who doesn't love a pair of cozy pajamas?

Pajama Pilates is a collection of these home exercises I've developed over the last 20 years of teaching, embellished with details and illustrations so that anyone can pick up this book and do the exercises safely.

Are you ready for Pajama Pilates? Let's get started!

GETTING STARTED

Pajama Pilates presents forty at-home exercises divided into four 10-to-15-minute exercise sets to do in your bedroom, kitchen, bathroom, and living room. You may do the exercises in sequence or choose your favorites in the order that feels right for your needs.

Complete with an introduction to basic Pilates concepts and key Pajama Pilates terms, these exercises are perfect for individuals at all levels. The bedroom set is suitable for beginners and can be used as a warm-up for the other, more challenging sets. I recommend doing these exercises daily, but please remember to listen to your body. If you need to start slow and build up to an everyday practice, that's OK too.

Each exercise includes simple, step-by-step instructions, a "Good for" section to highlight the physiological benefits, and a "Variations" section to explore the exercise in other ways or increase the difficulty. I also offer routines at the end to target common conditions or fitness goals my clients often come to me to address.

HERE'S ALL YOU NEED

→

Bed

Chair

Sofa

Table

Coffee table

Yoga mat or rug

Pillow

2 soup cans or light weights

Tennis ball

Towel

Bathtub

MY PAJAMA PILATES TIPS TO GET YOU STARTED

* Before starting, review the Five Basic Pilates Concepts on page 13 and Pajama Pilates Terms to Know on page 16.

* Try to exercise at the same time of day to establish a regular practice.

* Focus on your breath—inhale through your nose and exhale through your mouth.

* Maintain a slow and steady pace.

* Exhale on the exertion, or the part of the exercise that feels more difficult. This helps activate your core (see Core Activation on page 14) to support your movements.

* Listen to your body and move according to your abilities and within your limitations. Any suggested modifications are called out in the exercise.

* You can always increase the difficulty of the exercise by adding more repetitions. Gradually work up to more repetitions so you do not risk injury.

* In some variations, I recommend a certain number of reps, while in others, your body will tell you when it's time to stop.

* If you are pregnant, feel free to do side-lying, standing, or on-hands-and-knees exercises, but avoid exercises on your back or stomach.

* If you are injured, unwell, or recovering from surgery, ask your health practitioner if you can start a Pilates program.

FIVE BASIC PILATES CONCEPTS

These concepts are fundamental for Pilates. To have a safe and effective practice, it is important to remember these basics while performing each exercise in this book. As you move through the sets, refer back to this section every so often for a reminder. Eventually, they will become second nature to you.

1. Proper Body Alignment

A consistent Pilates practice will help you acquire the body awareness and the muscle memory necessary to find proper body alignment and to make adjustments on your own. Whether still or during movement, proper alignment prevents injuries and promotes healthy posture and body mechanics.

STANDING

You are in alignment if, standing sideways in front of a mirror, you can trace an imaginary plumb line that starts at the center of your ear and goes through the center of your shoulder, torso, hip, knee, and ankle in a straight line. When your head and shoulders slump forward or when your hips are farther forward than your shoulders, your body is not in alignment. To "stand tall," a cue used throughout this book to help you achieve standing alignment, shift your body weight toward your heels to equally distribute the weight between your two feet, hip distance apart. Then, imagine being pulled upward with a string from the crown of your head to lengthen your standing posture.

LYING DOWN

When lying on your back, you are in alignment when your shoulder blades and rib cage rest on the floor; your arms lie by your sides with your palms facing up, down, or in; and your spine is neutral (see Neutral Spine, page 15). To align your lower body, bend your knees, hip distance apart, so that your hip bones align with your knees. Place your feet flat on the floor with your weight equally distributed between them.

LEGS IN TABLETOP

When lying on your back, you are in alignment with legs in tabletop when your shoulder blades and rib cage rest on the floor; your arms lie by your sides with your palms facing up, down, or in; and your lumbar spine is imprinted (see Imprinted Lumbar

Spine on page 15). Your legs are lifted with your hips and knees both bent at 90 degrees so that your legs make a tabletop shape.

ON HANDS AND KNEES

When in this position, you are in alignment when your hands line up directly under your shoulders, your knees are directly under your hips, and your spine is in neutral. Your head is slightly lifted to create one long line from the top of your head to your tailbone, and your gaze is pointed toward the ground.

SIDE LYING

When in this position, you are in alignment if you are lying on your side with your shoulders and hips stacked and legs extended with a neutral spine.

2. Core Activation

The core is an ensemble of muscles in the center of the body that stabilize and protect your spine and pelvis from injury. *Core activation* is the motion of drawing in the deep abdominal muscles on an exhalation to turn the core on. In the book, I cue the visualization of "pulling the navel to the spine" to activate your core. This action causes a scooping of the lower belly—as if to hollow it out—to engage your deep abdominal muscles, creating intra-abdominal pressure. This takes weight off your spine and pelvis, making it easier to stabilize them, and the rest of your body, while you are in motion.

3. Neutral Spine

A *neutral spine* specifically refers to the natural concave curve of your lumbar spine (the lower back), and most exercises in this book are done with a neutral spine. Explore finding your neutral spine by standing sideways in front of a mirror and tucking your tailbone, then do the opposite and overexaggerate the curve by sticking your tailbone out. You'll notice neither one of these positions has the natural curve of a neutral spine, but by neither tucking nor jutting your tailbone, you maintain a stabilized pelvis, which allows you to find a neutral spine. Another way to explore this concept is to lie down relaxed on your back and feel the space between your lumbar spine and the ground—the size of which varies from person to person—this is your spine in neutral.

4. Imprinted Lumbar Spine

You have an *imprinted lumbar spine* when you lie on your back and activate your core to flatten your lumbar spine to the ground, closing the space formed by your neutral spine. To imprint your lumbar spine, activate your core by pulling your navel to your spine and slightly tilting your pelvis upward. This is important in some exercises, like the ones with your legs in tabletop position, to protect your lower back.

5. Stabilizer Muscles

For all movements of the body, there are primary muscles that are the big movers performing the action, such as the glutes and quads in a squat, and other muscles that stabilize and support them, ensuring your body structure stays intact. The core is a big stabilizer of the spine and pelvis; we also have stabilizer muscles at each joint that help keep them in place and free from injury.

PAJAMA PILATES
TERMS TO KNOW

These are terms I use often throughout the book.
Familiarize yourself with them and you will be a pro in no time.

CORE MUSCLES

Also called *powerhouse*, *inner unit*, or *deep abdominals*, the core is an ensemble of muscles in the center of our body organized in a cylindrical shape. At the top is the diaphragm; at the bottom the pelvic floor; and the middle muscles include the transversus abdominis (or TA), the quadratus lumborum, the internal obliques, the psoas major, and the multifidi in the spine. Learning how to activate the core properly is the main focus in Pilates, and the key to providing stability to all movements, protecting the spine and pelvis, and preventing injuries.

EXTENSOR AND FLEXOR MUSCLES

These muscles perform extensions and flexions in the body. For example, in the arm, an extensor muscle is the triceps and a flexor muscle is the biceps. The triceps extends, or straightens, the arm and the biceps flexes, or bends, the arm.

FASCIA

This soft connective tissue under the skin is densely interlaced like a spiderweb and extends throughout the body, enclosing and holding everything together. Some movements and stretches in this book will revive and restore the fascia in different parts of the body.

GLUTEAL MUSCLES

The gluteals, or "glutes" for short, are hip extensors; they are the large muscles of the buttocks and the hips that, among other things, activate to help move from squatting or sitting to standing upright.

HAMSTRING

This muscle, located in the back of the thigh between the hip and the knee, among other functions, bends the knees and helps extend the hips to bring the leg behind the body, critical for walking and running. The hamstrings can get tight and pull on the lower back, causing discomfort.

HIP ABDUCTORS AND ADDUCTORS

The abductor muscles are located in the outer thigh and pull the leg away from the midline (see Midline, right). The adductor muscles, located in the inner thigh, pull the leg toward the midline.

HIP FLEXORS

This muscle group flexes at the hip and allows the thigh to lift toward the chest. Psoas major is one of the strongest of the hip flexors. Due to our sedentary lifestyle, it's very common to have a tight psoas muscle—its symptoms are tension and pain in the lower back and hips.

LATISSIMUS DORSI

Known as the "lats," these triangular-shaped muscles connect the upper arm to the spine. They have a key role in moving and stabilizing the shoulder and rotating, extending, and side-bending the upper torso.

MIDLINE

This is an imaginary center line that divides the body equally between the left and right sides.

OBLIQUES

The obliques are abdominal muscles, both internal and external, that wrap around the rib cage and provide stability to the spine while flexing and rotating the upper body.

PELVIS

Made up of four big bones, the sacrum, the tailbone, and hip bones on each side, the pelvis connects the spine with the lower limbs and protects the abdominal organs.

PULSES

These are small, fast movements up and down or side to side in a limited range of motion.

RIB CAGE

A system of bones (the ribs) connects the spine to the sternum to protect the lungs and heart. If you put your hands around your rib cage and take a breath, you can feel the ribs expanding out.

SACROILIAC JOINT

The sacroiliac joint, or SI for short, is where the sacrum connects with the hip bones of the pelvis. There are two of them, one on each side. When the SI joint is unstable, you may experience pain typically at the very top of the sacrum on one or both sides.

SACRUM

A large, upside-down triangle bone, the sacrum is the base of the spine. Its bottom point is fused to the coccyx, or tailbone. Together with the two hip bones, it forms the pelvis.

SCAPULA (PLURAL: *SCAPULAE*)

The scapula, also known as the shoulder blade, is a flat triangular bone that sits on one side of your upper back. You have a scapula on each side of your back, like wings, that connects to both your collar-bone and upper arm bone (the humerus). Scapulae are very mobile bones that can move up and down, forward and back, and protract and retract from each other (see Shoulder Blade Isolation on page 27).

SIT BONES

These are the two bones you sit on that form the lower part of your pelvis. When you sit up straight, you are balancing on your sit bones.

SPINE

The spine, or backbone, extends from the base of the skull to the tailbone and is made of thirty-three bones, called *verte-brae*. The segments of the spine are: cervical (neck), thoracic (chest), lumbar (lower back), sacrum (see Sacrum, page 18), and coccyx (tailbone). Developing a healthy core will stabilize and protect the spine.

SPINE EXTENSORS

This group of muscles runs the length of the spine on both sides, from the sacrum to the base of the skull. They allow the spine to extend and help keep correct posture.

STEP

A "step" in Pajama Pilates is measured by the distance of your natural stride; its length varies from person to person.

IN THE

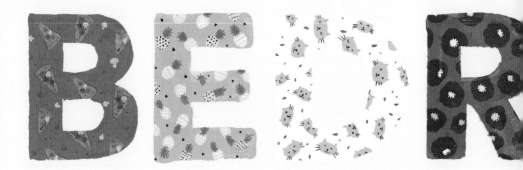

BE OR

Rise and shine! Or, as the old Italian proverb goes,
"Chi dorme non piglia pesci!" (Roughly meaning, "You won't
catch any fish while you're asleep.") These exercises help
you gently wake up and prepare your body to meet the day.

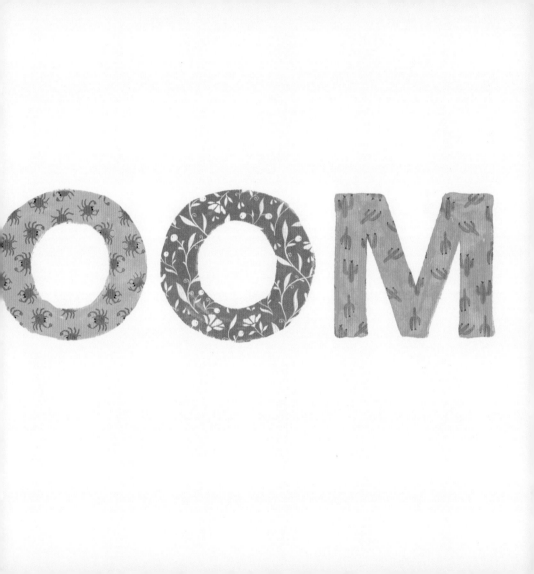

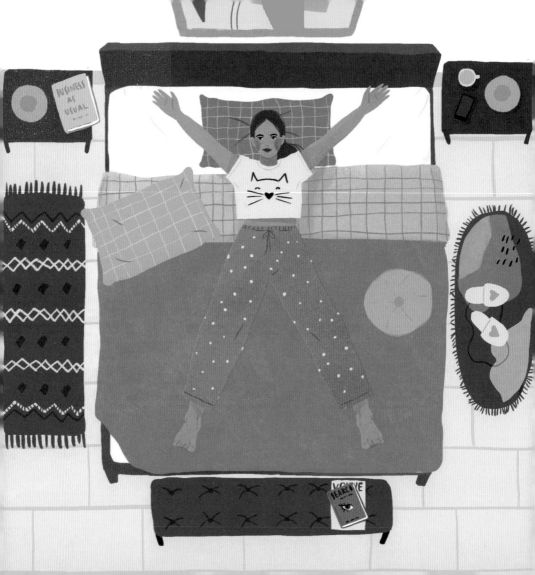

THE STAR

The Star revives and loosens up your fascia and gets your body ready to move. The word *pandiculate* describes stretching, yawning, and releasing, much the way a dog or a cat does. So...let's pandiculate!

GOOD FOR

Releasing the fascia in the front of the body; activating the core; improving flexibility

VARIATION

You can do this throughout the day, standing or sitting at your desk.

1 Lie on your back.

2 As you inhale, stretch your arms over your head and reach your legs out toward the four corners of the bed so that you mimic the shape of a star. Face your palms up and point your feet while you are stretching. Hold briefly.

3 Exhale as you relax into the bed. Pause.

4 Repeat, completing 3 to 5 reps.

INHALE-EXHALE

Our breath connects our body and mind, helping us calm down. Healthy breathing improves brain function, energy level, and muscle performance. Activating the breathing muscles, especially the diaphragm, abdominals, and rib-cage muscles, is essential in Pilates and life.

GOOD FOR

Connecting body and mind; decreasing stress; releasing tension in the neck and shoulders; opening the chest; improving lung capacity; activating the core

VARIATION

As you exhale, pull your navel to your spine to imprint your lumbar spine. As you inhale, return to a neutral spine.

1 Lie on your back with proper body alignment.

2 Inhale through your nose, allowing the air you take in to expand your rib cage in all directions.

3 Exhale through your mouth. As you exhale, notice a light activation of your core.

4 Repeat, completing 10 to 15 reps.

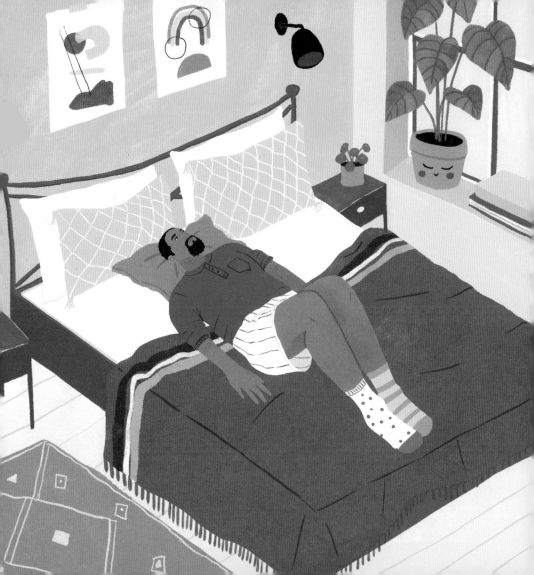

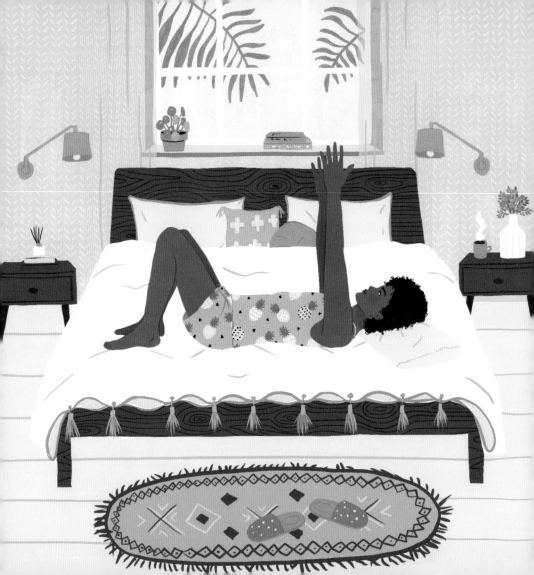

SHOULDER BLADE
ISOLATION

In this exercise, you are focusing on isolating the shoulder blades (scapulae) and activating their stabilizing muscles. Because the shoulder is one of the most mobile, and also unstable, joints in the body, these supportive muscles must work together to keep the scapulae in place.

GOOD FOR

Opening the chest; activating the core and shoulder stabilizer muscles

VARIATIONS

Alternate sides, reaching one arm up and isolating one shoulder blade at a time.

Hold light weights while you do the exercise.

1 Lie on your back with your arms reaching up over your shoulders, palms facing in, knees bent, feet flat on the bed, and legs parallel and hip distance apart.

2 Reach toward the ceiling with your fingertips as you simultaneously glide the scapulae apart. This movement is subtle, but you should feel a stretch between your shoulders.

3 Bring your scapulae back to the starting position to feel the shoulder stabilizer muscles activating.

4 Repeat, completing 10 reps.

GENTLE PELVIC TILT

Your lower back was still all night; this is the stretch it deserves. At first it may feel a bit stiff, but as you move, it will loosen up. Motion is lotion!

GOOD FOR

Activating the core; strengthening the glutes and hamstrings; increasing spine flexibility

VARIATION

Hold your tailbone up off the bed for 3 to 5 breaths.

1 Lie on your back with proper body alignment.

2 Press the soles of your feet into the bed to activate your glutes.

3 Pull your navel to your spine and tuck your tailbone to tilt your pelvis and lift it slightly off the bed.

4 Slowly return to the starting position.

5 Repeat, completing 10 reps.

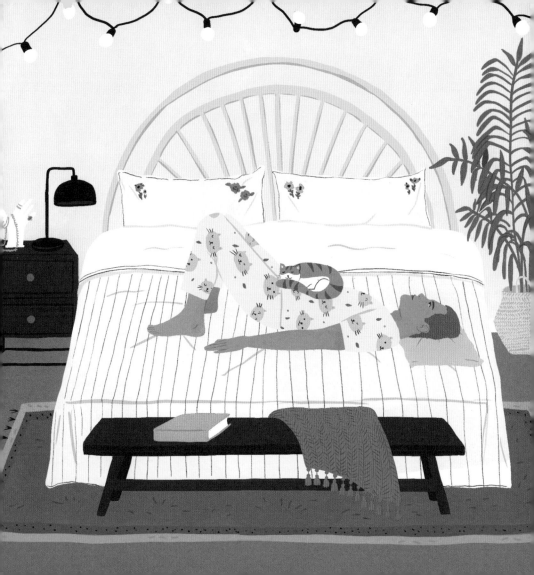

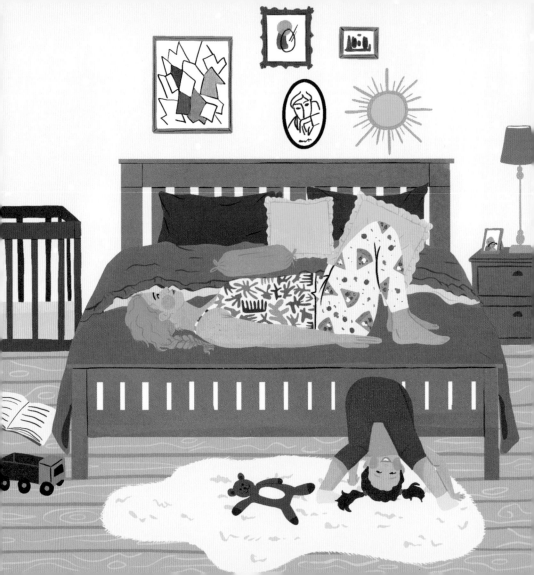

PILLOW SQUEEZE

A good way to visualize this exercise, which activates the core and strengthens your adductor muscles, or inner thigh muscles, is to think of zipping your inner thighs together from your knees to your hips while you squeeze a pillow between them. Activating your adductors will make your core spark.

GOOD FOR

Strengthening the adductor muscles; activating the core; stabilizing the lower back and pelvis; aligning the SI joint

VARIATION

Alternate legs, using just one thigh to press the pillow, then the other. That's 1 rep. Repeat, completing 10 reps.

1 Lie on your back with proper body alignment. Place a pillow between your legs.

2 Squeeze the pillow with your thighs for the duration of your exhaling breath, keeping your glutes relaxed.

3 As you inhale, release the squeeze.

4 Repeat, completing 10 reps.

SINGLE-SIDED LEG LIFT

It's time for a little more core activation with the Single-Sided Leg Lift. Get your core ready to wake up along with you.

GOOD FOR

Activating the core; strengthening the hip flexors; stabilizing the spine and pelvis

VARIATION

Raise both legs to tabletop. Lower and lift one leg and then the other. That's 1 rep. Repeat, completing 10 reps.

1 Lie on your back with proper body alignment.

2 Pull your navel to your spine and lift your right leg to tabletop position, with your hip and knee each bent at a 90-degree angle.

3 Lower your leg 45 degrees to feel a core activation.

4 Return your leg to tabletop position.

5 Repeat, completing 10 reps, then switch, completing 10 reps on your left leg.

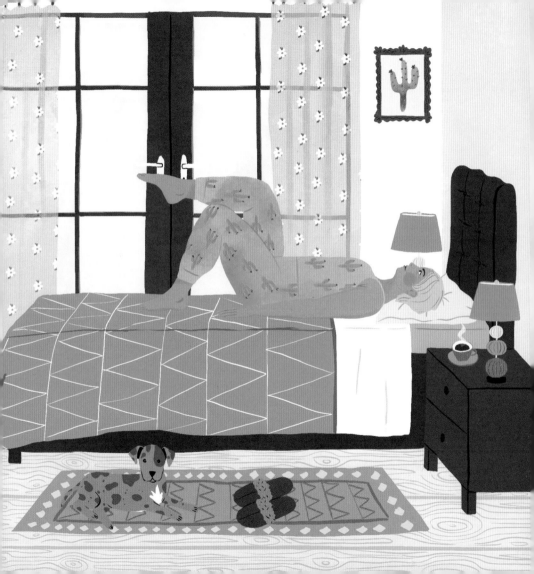

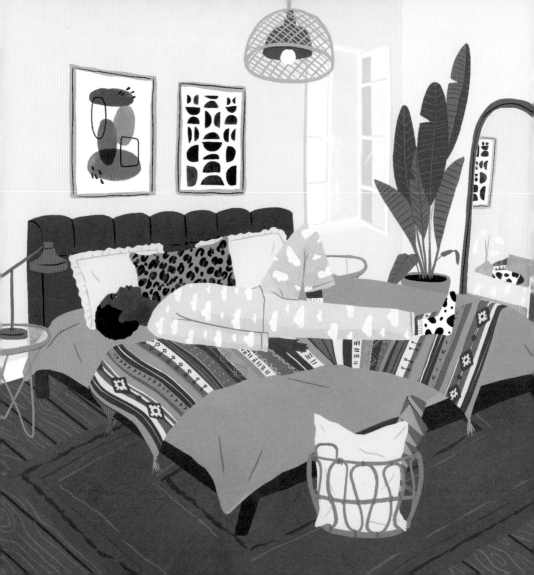

SINGLE-SIDED LEG SLIDE

As you slide your leg, imagine you have a cup of water sitting on your belly. If you can balance it without spilling, your pelvis is stabilized. This exercise is like a spa treatment for your hips; and, as the song says, your hips don't lie.

GOOD FOR

Strengthening the hip flexors; increasing hip mobility; activating the core; stabilizing the pelvis

VARIATION

Slide both legs together at the same time.

1 Lie on your back with proper body alignment.

2 Extend one leg, sliding your heel away from your hip until your leg is straight—while keeping your pelvis stable.

3 Slide your leg back to the starting position.

4 Repeat, completing 10 reps, then switch, completing 10 reps on the other side.

TABLETOP HOLD

If you have not really felt your core activate just yet, this will be the moment!

Activating the core; strengthening the hip flexors

Extend both legs straight toward the ceiling, then bring your legs to tabletop position. Repeat, completing 5 to 10 reps.

1 Lie on your back with proper body alignment.

2 Pull your navel to your spine, imprinting your lumbar spine.

3 Bring one leg at a time to tabletop position. Hold this position for 3 complete inhale-exhale breaths (see page 24).

4 One at a time, bring your legs down to the bed.

5 Repeat, completing 3 to 5 reps.

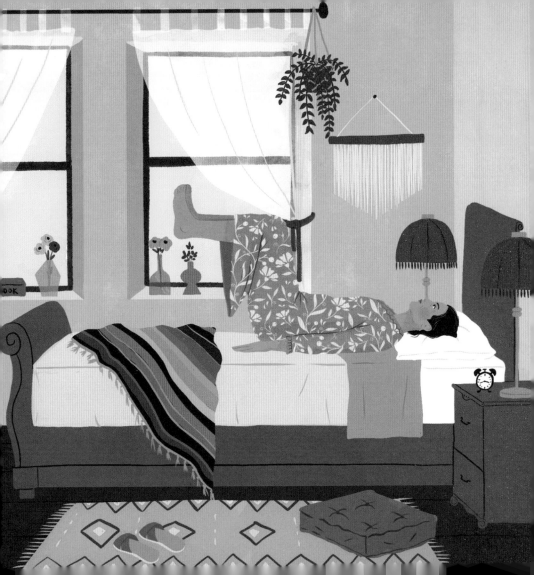

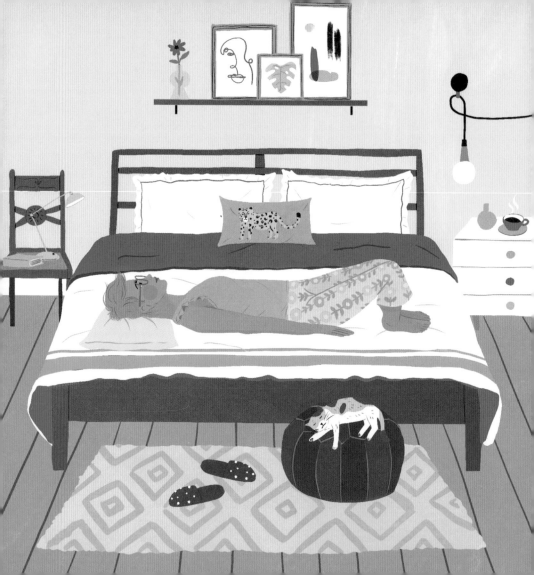

WINDSHIELD WIPER KNEES

Here's some exciting action for your obliques and, of course, your core. A common mistake with Windshield Wiper Knees is to rely on your quads to assist; to get the most benefit and challenge, focus on isolating your movements to just your core muscles.

GOOD FOR

Strengthening the obliques; stabilizing the spine and pelvis; activating the core

VARIATION

Start with your legs in tabletop position and sway your knees to one side and then the other.

1 Lie on your back with proper body alignment.

2 Pull your navel to your spine, imprinting your lumbar spine.

3 Now sway your knees, first to one side and then to the other, keeping your head, shoulders, and ribs on the bed; you may lift the opposite hip slightly off the bed.

4 Repeat, completing 5 reps.

ONE-LEG CIRCLE

Have you ever felt that one side of your body moves better than the other? As if one side is floating in water, while the other side is moving through mud? Imbalances in the body are common because we each have one dominant side that is used more than the other. Pilates focuses on creating balance and strengthening both sides of your body equally.

GOOD FOR

Stabilizing the hip, pelvis, and spine; activating the core; strengthening the hip flexors

VARIATION

Straighten your leg toward the ceiling and then perform the repetitions, creating larger circles while continuing to stabilize your pelvis.

1 Lie on your back with proper body alignment.

2 Lift one leg to tabletop position, keeping your knee bent and your foot flexed.

3 Make small circles at the hip joint while keeping your pelvis stable.

4 Repeat, completing 5 reps clockwise and 5 reps counterclockwise, then switch, completing 5 reps clockwise and 5 reps counterclockwise on the other side.

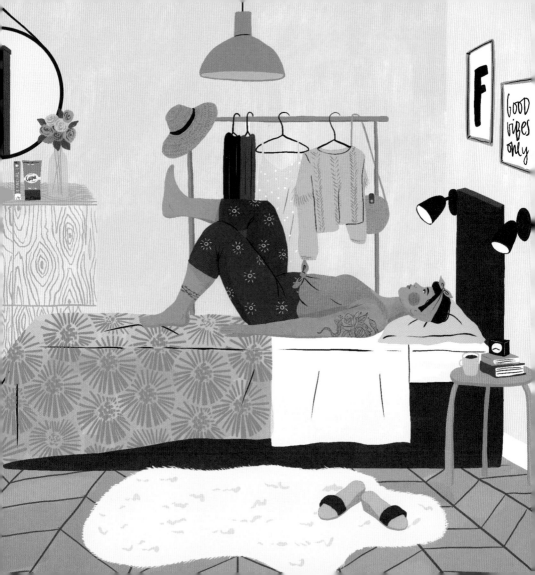

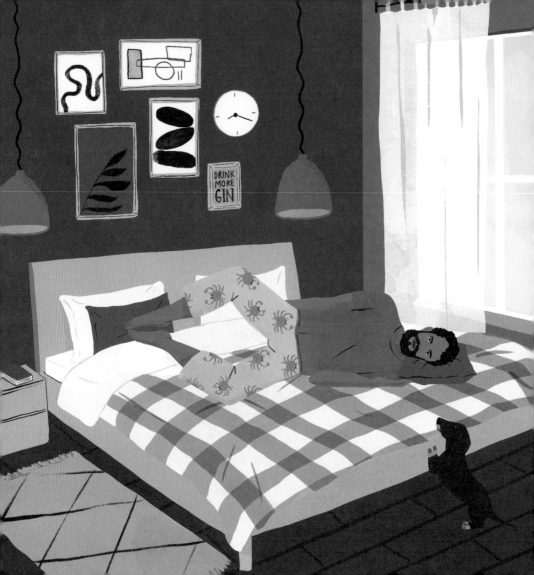

SIDE-LYING CLAM SHELL

The Side-Lying Clam Shell engages a range of muscles, including muscles in your core, hips, and back. Many physical therapists I know use it as a strengthening cure-all because it targets several areas at once.

GOOD FOR

Activating the core; strengthening the abductors and glutes; increasing hip mobility; stabilizing the hip and spine; improving balance

VARIATION

Place your top hand against your thigh, providing some resistance for your knee to push against as it lifts.

1 Lie on your side with proper body alignment, supporting your head with a pillow. Rest your bottom arm on the bed and your top arm on your side.

2 Bend your knees at about 45 degrees with your legs together.

3 Lift both feet slightly off the bed and keep them elevated throughout the exercise.

4 Lift your top knee with a spiral movement from your hip joint, keeping your feet together, like a clam opening its shell. Then, lower your raised knee, closing the "clam shell."

5 Repeat, completing 10 reps, then switch, completing 10 reps on the other side.

SIDE-LYING SPINE TWIST

And now, it's time for a well-deserved stretch to open your chest and loosen your shoulders. Keep a soup can handy for the variation.

GOOD FOR

Stretching the obliques, chest, and front of shoulder; stabilizing the hips; activating the core

VARIATION

Hold a soup can or a light weight in the hand of your upper arm (the arm that rotates).

1 Lie on your side with proper body alignment. Bend your hips and knees to about 90 degrees with your arms forward, resting on the bed, palms together and raised to shoulder level.

2 As you inhale, fan open your upper arm and rotate your chest to open toward the ceiling, allowing your upper body to gently twist while your hips remain sideways and your arms spread out into the shape of a *T*.

3 Keep your fanned arm at shoulder level and hold the position for 3 breaths. Then return to the starting position.

4 Repeat, completing 3 reps, then switch, completing 3 reps on the other side.

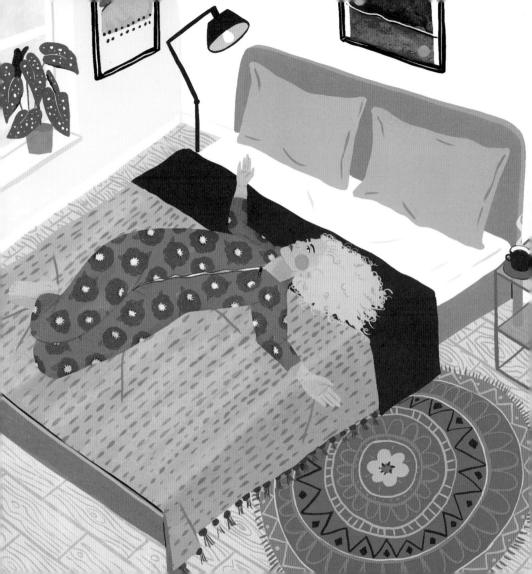

IN THE

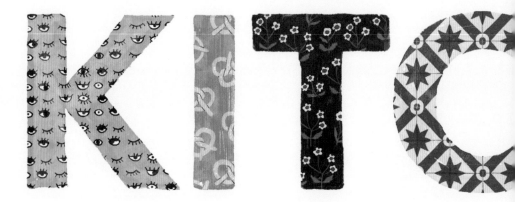

KITC

Now let's go to the kitchen; it's time for coffee and tea!
While you are waiting for your brew, with its aroma
enveloping you, keep moving and challenge your core.
You will need a towel and a counter or a sturdy table.

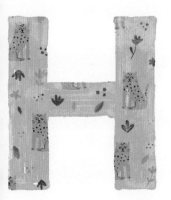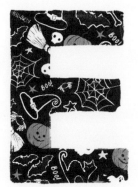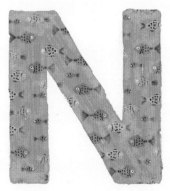

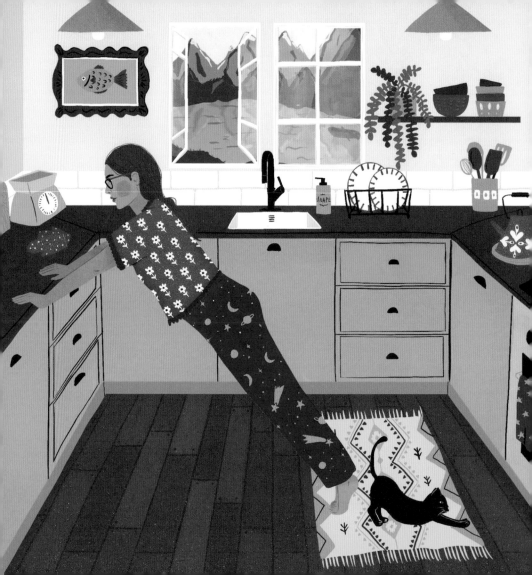

STANDING PLANK

Whether you are a runner, hiker, gardener, or golfer, simply holding this position for as long as you can while still keeping proper body alignment will make your core stronger. You will know when it's time to rest! If your wrists hurt in this position, try leaning on your forearms instead of your hands. Add a folded towel under your arms to make it more comfy.

GOOD FOR

Strengthening the obliques, hip adductors, glutes, quads, and hamstrings; stabilizing the shoulders; activating the core; promoting good posture; improving stamina

VARIATIONS

Increase your time in the plank.

Alternate hovering one leg off the ground in the plank.

1 Stand tall 2 to 3 steps away from the kitchen counter, far enough that you can lean forward with your arms straight out in front of you to grasp the counter edge.

2 Line up your body so that your shoulders, ribs, hips, knees, and feet are all in alignment—as if one straight line connects your head to your feet—while gently drawing your shoulders down, away from your ears. You are now in the plank position.

3 Hold the plank for 10 to 30 seconds. Then return to an upright position.

4 Repeat, completing 3 to 5 reps.

BALANCING
BACK LEG LIFT

If you sit at a desk daily for an extended period, you are at risk of tightened hip flexors, joint misalignment, and weakening glute muscles, all of which can lead to lower back pain. This exercise will help you counter some of the negative effects of sitting day in and day out.

GOOD FOR

Strengthening the glutes, chest, and back muscles; improving hip mobility and balance; preventing falls

VARIATIONS

Point and flex your raised foot.

While your leg is raised, pulse it up and down.

1 Stand tall 1 step away from the kitchen counter so your straight arms reach the edge of the counter or table.

2 Hinge forward at your hips with a straight back, bending your elbows back. Simultaneously, lift one leg straight back and bring your chest toward the counter, keeping your head and leg in alignment and your hips parallel to the ground.

3 Return to a standing position as you straighten your arms, bring your chest up, and lower your leg to the ground.

4 Repeat, completing 10 to 20 reps, then switch, completing 10 to 20 reps on the other side.

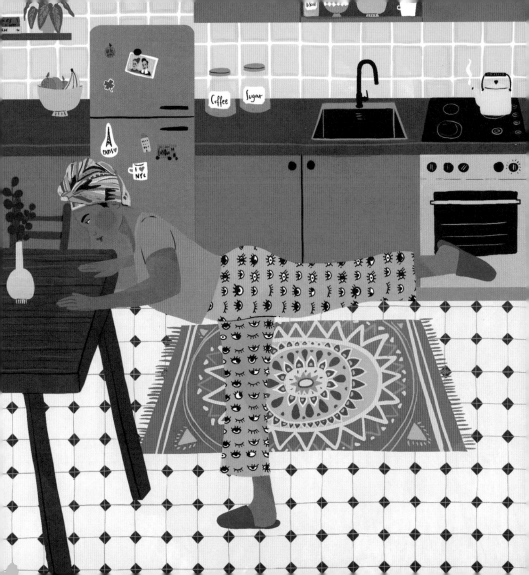

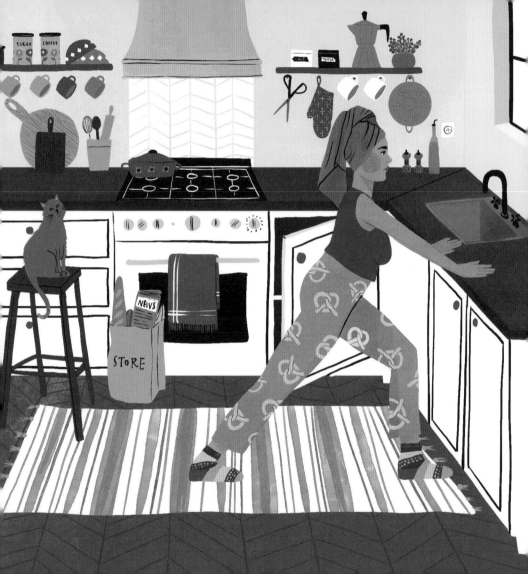

CALF STRETCH

You will find this stretch so satisfying after a walk, hike, or run; it helps avoid the tightening of your calf and ankle muscles.

GOOD FOR

Improving ankle and foot mobility; improving calf muscle flexibility

VARIATION

Slightly bend your back knee to feel the stretch moving in the lower part of your calf.

1 Facing the counter, place one leg 1 step away from the counter and the other leg 2 steps away from the counter. Then bend your front knee, keeping the back leg straight.

2 Hold this position, keeping your back heel down on the floor to feel a stretch in the calf of your back leg.

3 Breathe into the stretch for 30 to 60 seconds.

4 Repeat on the opposite leg.

TABLE STRETCH

You can do this stretch anywhere—at home, work, school, a friend's house. No, really! It's a great stress release and helps you regroup and re-center after staring at a screen for many hours.

GOOD FOR

Stretching the shoulders, hips, glutes, hamstrings, and calves; restoring the fascia; relaxing the body and calming the mind

VARIATIONS

Open your arms wider to move the stretch to another spot in the chest or shoulders.

Move both arms to the same side of the table and breathe into your ribs on the opposite side of your body, lengthening and creating more space in between each rib bone.

1 Stand tall away from a counter or a sturdy table so your arms fully extend to reach the surface edge.

2 Hinge at the hips with a straight back, letting your resting hands and forearms equally support your weight.

3 Breathe, expanding your rib cage in all directions.

4 Hold this position for as long as it feels good.

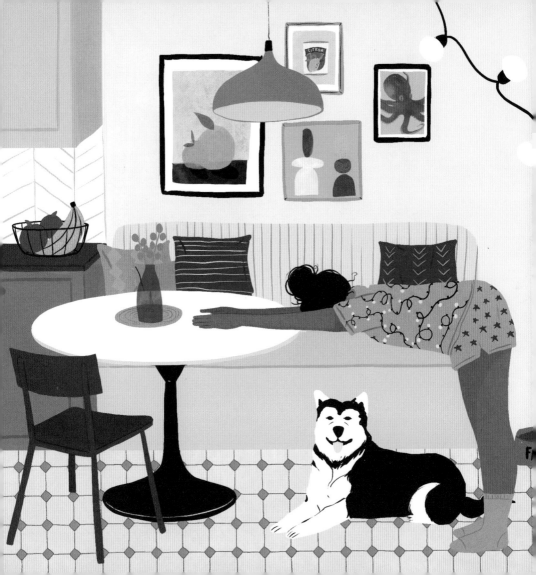

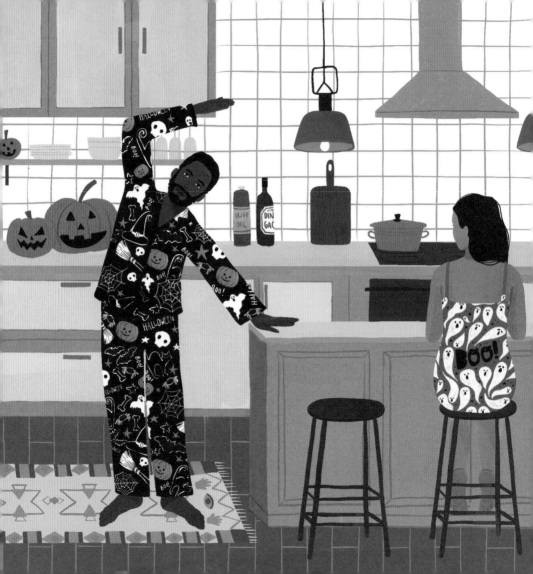

KITCHEN COUNTER SIDE BEND

One of my clients, an anesthesiologist who spends most of her work day hovering over patients and bending and twisting her upper body, does the Kitchen Counter Side Bend a few times a day to expand her rib cage, create space between her ribs and her hips, and feel a nice release in her sides.

GOOD FOR

Restoring the fascia; improving rib mobility; stretching the obliques, lats, and lower back

VARIATION

Turn your chest and lifted arm toward the counter to feel a deeper stretch in the back of the shoulder.

1 Stand tall sideways next to a counter or table, placing one hand on it and lifting your other arm overhead.

2 Bend sideways toward the counter, feeling a stretch through your lifted arm side.

3 Hold this position for 3 full breaths, keeping both feet planted firmly.

4 Repeat, completing 3 reps, then switch, completing 3 reps on the other side.

TEXT NECK CHEST OPENER

If the bad posture caused by texting or staring at a screen (termed "Text Neck" by Dr. D. L. Fishman)—which includes a tilted neck, tight chest, and weak upper back muscles—were a poison, this exercise would be its antidote. You can do this exercise while waiting for your coffee or even on a work break.

Improving posture; opening the chest; strengthening the upper spine extensors

Bring one arm at a time overhead as you are opening the chest.

Interlace your fingers behind your body, squeezing your shoulder blades together to expand your chest.

1 Stand tall at a counter with your feet parallel, hip distance apart, and your body weight equally distributed on both feet.

2 Keeping your chin down, press your hands onto the counter and tilt the bottom of your shoulder blades forward and upward so your chest is pointing toward the ceiling and there is a slight arch in your upper back.

3 Return to your starting position.

4 Repeat, completing 5 to 8 reps.

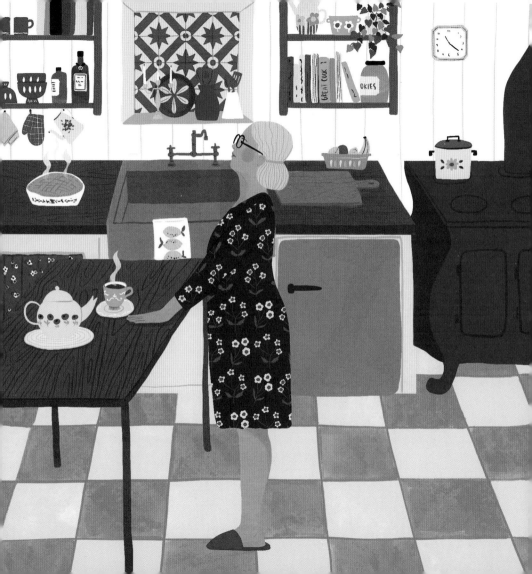

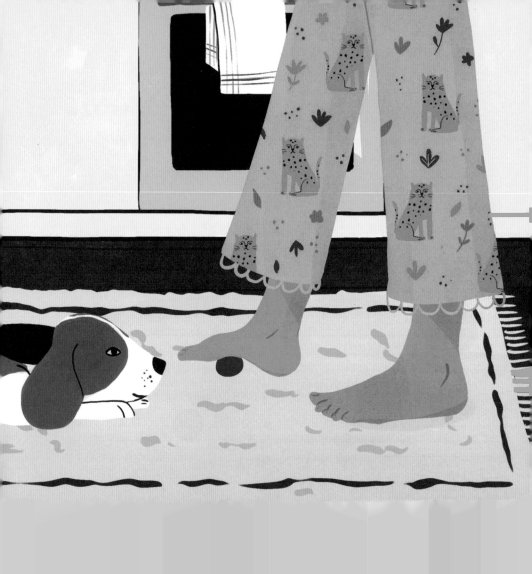

TENNIS BALL FOOT ROLL

Here's a chance to show your feet some gratitude. This exercise benefits the 26 bones, 33 joints, and more than 100 muscles, tendons, and ligaments found in your foot. Have a tennis ball close by for this one.

GOOD FOR

Restoring the plantar (foot) fascia; strengthening the ankle and foot muscles; improving balance

VARIATIONS

With your heel on the floor and the ball under the ball of your foot, shift your weight onto the ball of your foot to squish the ball. Then gently release the pressure by bringing the weight back.

With your heel on the floor and the ball under the ball of your foot, twist your foot from side to side.

1 Stand on one foot, holding on to a counter or sturdy table.

2 Place your raised foot on top of a tennis ball. Roll your foot up and down on the ball while applying light pressure for about 30 seconds.

3 Repeat on the opposite foot.

SEATED FIGURE FOUR

Let's bring our attention to our hips. One of the six hip rotators, the piriformis is a flat, bandlike muscle located in the buttocks area. It runs parallel to the sciatic nerve; when it is tight and inflamed, people may experience sciatica. You may also feel tightness after a long flight or sitting in the car on a road trip. I have not met anyone who does not like this stretch!

GOOD FOR

Stretching the piriformis and hip muscles; providing relief from sciatica

VARIATION

You can do the same stretch lying on your back on the floor.

1 Sit at the edge of a chair, with your weight equally distributed on both sit bones and your feet flat on the floor.

2 Cross one leg over the other, with the ankle of the crossed leg resting on your thigh and your bent knee pointing away from your midline, creating the number four with your legs.

3 Hinge your upper torso forward to bend slightly at the hips and hold the stretch for 30 seconds.

4 Repeat, completing the stretch on the other side.

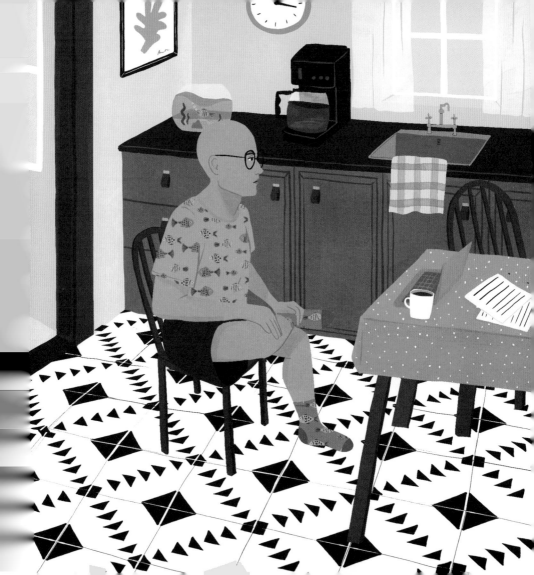

IN THE

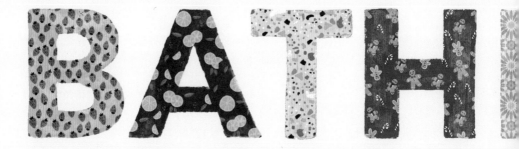

BATHI

Now it's time to get ready for the day, but why
stop challenging your body? Keep on moving!
You will need a towel and a pillow handy.

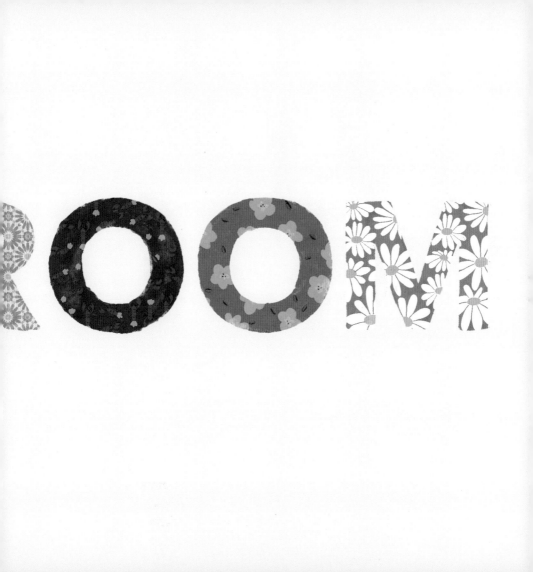

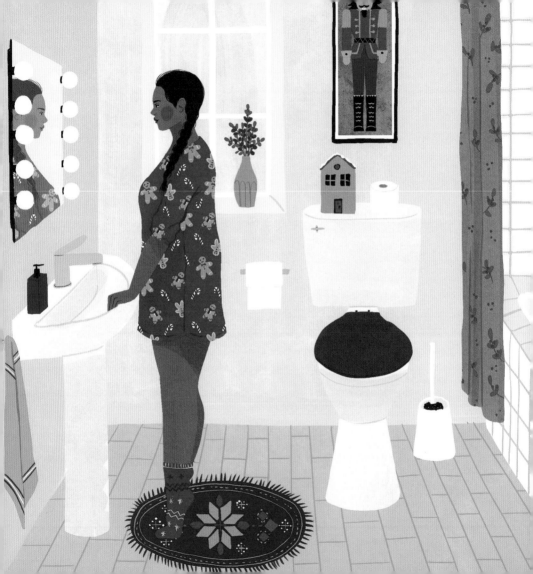

STANDING HEEL RAISE

Let's rise up using the power of our calf muscles to balance on our toes and the balls of our feet. This strengthens our ankles and feet, improving our balance.

GOOD FOR

Activating the core; improving ankle mobility and strength; improving balance; strengthening the calf muscles and glutes

VARIATIONS

On tiptoe, lower one heel and bend the opposite knee. Alternate to your other heel and opposite knee. That's 1 rep. Repeat, completing 20 to 30 reps.

Raise one foot. Lift and then lower the heel of your other foot. Repeat, completing 10 to 15 reps on each side.

1 Stand tall with your feet parallel, distributing your weight equally on both feet and pressing your weight into both big toes. Hold the sink with your hands.

2 Lift both heels and stand on tiptoe, with your weight on your toes and the balls of your feet, for 1 to 2 breaths or as long you can keep your balance. Lower your heels back to the floor.

3 Repeat, completing 10 to 20 reps.

ONE-FOOT BALANCING ACT

Balance while brushing your teeth: It's a twofer, or shall I say a "toother"? Do one, get one free. Practice this every day and you will strengthen your hips, knees, and ankles, and will also be steadier on your feet. The name is an homage to my circus days!

GOOD FOR

Strengthening the glutes and ankle muscles; improving balance; preventing falls (bonus: sparkling teeth!)

VARIATIONS

Lift the arm opposite your raised leg to the ceiling; then alternate your arm when you switch your leg.

Lift and lower the heel of your planted foot.

1 While brushing your teeth, lift one leg. Shift your weight to your planted foot, feeling your hip and leg muscles activating. Hold the counter for balance if needed.

2 Keep your leg elevated for 30 to 60 seconds, then lower your leg back to the ground

3 Repeat on the other side.

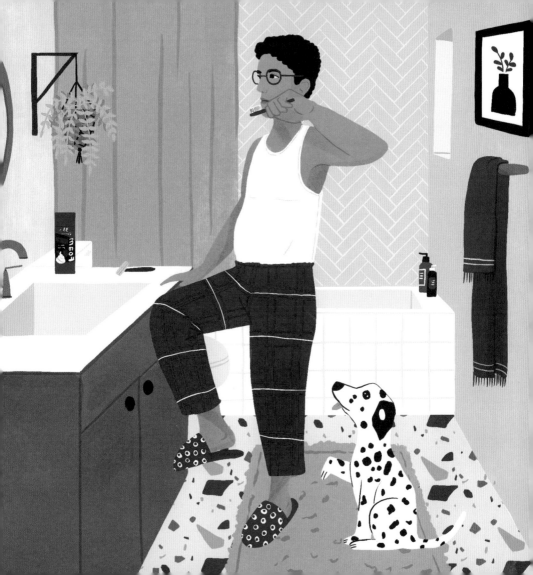

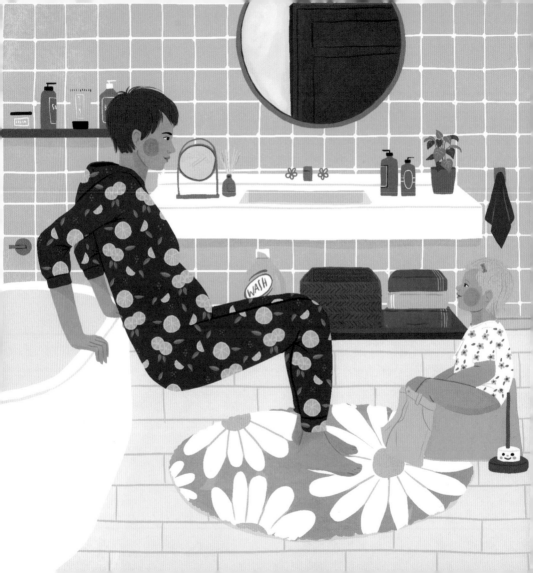

BATHTUB TRICEPS DIP

That's right, the bathtub! It can be used for exercising. Triceps dips will tone the back of your arms—and who doesn't like defined triceps! This is the go-to exercise for upper body strength. If you do not have a bathtub, try this on the edge of a sturdy chair or coffee table.

GOOD FOR

Strengthening the triceps; activating the core and shoulder stabilizer muscles

VARIATIONS

Walk your feet out farther and perform the dips with straight legs instead of bending them at 90 degrees.

Add up and down pulses.

Now combine the two previous variations: Straighten your legs and add pulses. You'll thank me later!

1 Stand tall, facing away from the tub. Take 1 step away and bring your arms behind your body. Bend your knees and place your hands on the edge of the tub with your palms down and fingers pointed outside the tub.

2 Walk your feet out another step away so your knees are bent about 90 degrees.

3 Bend your elbows, lowering your hips toward the ground until your elbows are bent about 90 degrees.

4 Straighten your arms to slowly push yourself back to the starting position.

5 Repeat, completing 10 to 15 reps.

SINK SQUAT

Both Moscow and Mexico City came up with an imaginative way to keep their populations fit and healthy: They asked commuters to do squats in exchange for a free subway ticket. You can do this too, but in your pajamas holding on to your sink. Keep two soup cans or light weights handy for the variation.

GOOD FOR

Activating the core; strengthening the quads, glutes, hamstrings, and lats; improving ankle, knee, and hip joint mobility

VARIATIONS

Add up and down pulses in the squat position.

Hold soup cans or weights in your hands and bring your arms forward with your palms facing in as you squat.

1 Stand tall facing the sink about half a step away. Hold on to the edge of the sink.

2 Bend your knees to 90 degrees, as if sitting on a chair, slightly hinging forward at the hips while keeping a neutral spine.

3 Return to the starting position by pressing your heels into the floor as you straighten your legs; you should feel your buttock muscles activating.

4 Repeat, completing 10 to 30 reps.

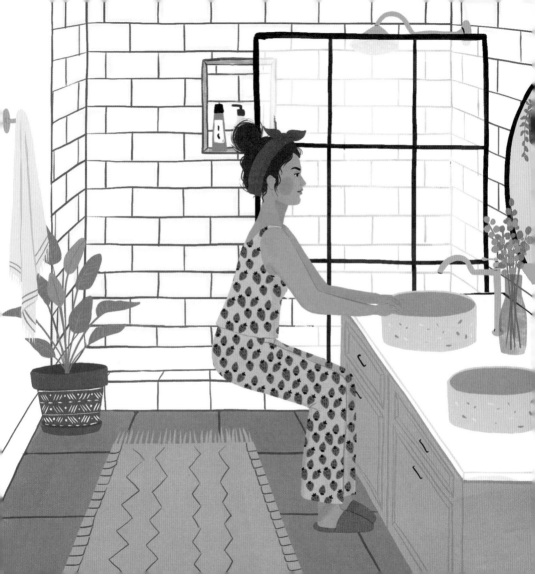

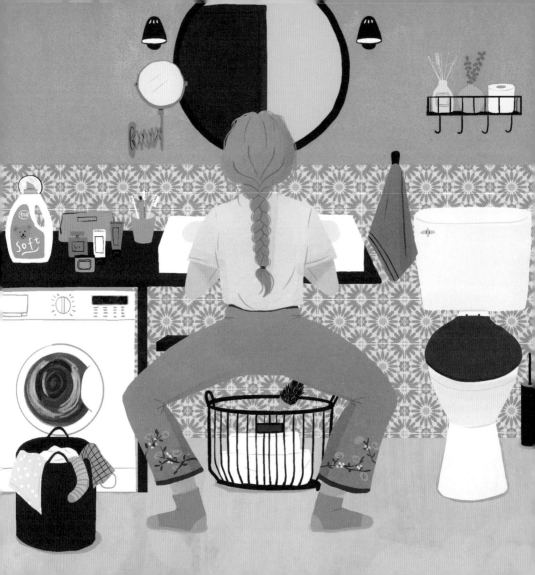

GRAND PLIÉ

This exercise is based on a foundational pose in ballet that I often use in my client sessions. Imagine a soft piano playing in the background as if you are training to become a ballet dancer. This may even inspire smoother and more graceful movements!

GOOD FOR

Strengthening the glutes, quads, hamstrings, and adductors (inner thigh muscles); improving balance

VARIATIONS

Bring your arms forward as you plié.

As your balance improves, bring your arms above your head as you plié.

1 Stand tall, with your legs spread apart wider than hip distance and toes pointed forward; hold the edge of the sink for balance.

2 Open your hips by rotating your legs so that your knees and toes point outward 45 degrees from your midline.

3 Keeping your feet firmly planted on the ground, bend your knees to about 90 degrees, making sure your knees line up with your toes and your spine is neutral.

4 Straighten your legs back to the starting position.

5 Repeat, completing 10 to 20 reps.

ALTERNATING ARM AND LEG REACH

If you would like to strengthen your lower back, this is a good exercise for you. People who have tender wrists can perform this exercise with forearms and bent elbows resting on a folded towel on the edge of the tub. If your bathroom is cramped, save this exercise for the living room floor.

GOOD FOR

Activating the core, shoulder, spine, and hip stabilizer muscles; strengthening the glutes

VARIATIONS

Hold the position for 2 or 3 breaths.

Add up and down leg pulses while continuing to maintain proper hip alignment.

1 Find your on-hands-and-knees position with proper body alignment. Pull your navel to the spine to activate your core, and direct your gaze toward the ground.

2 Using your core strength, extend one arm forward, palm facing in, as you simultaneously reach your opposite leg back. Keep your hips level and avoid shifting your weight from side to side.

3 Return your extended arm and leg to the on-hands-and-knees position.

4 Repeat, completing 3 to 5 reps, then switch, completing 3 to 5 reps with the opposite arm and leg.

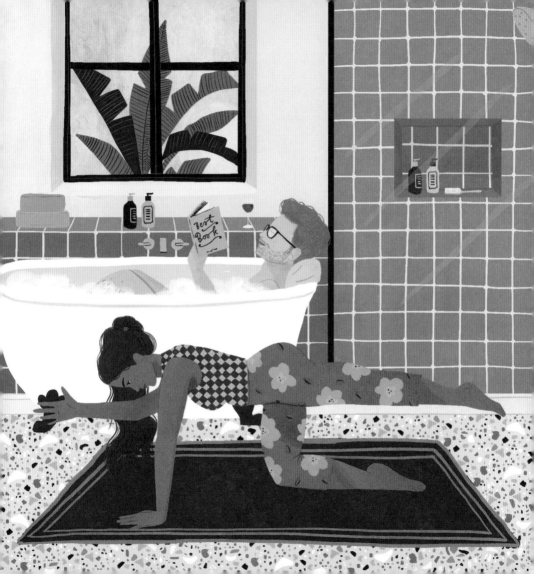

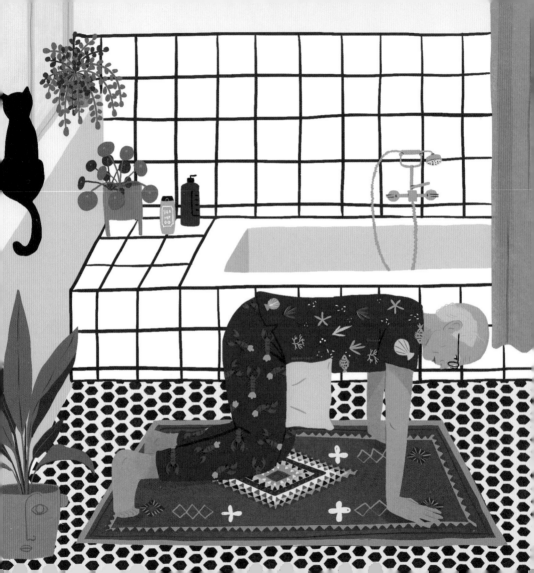

DOUBLE KNEE LIFT

This exercise may look easy to do, but in fact it's quite challenging! You may feel your heart racing and your muscles shaking if you hold it for long enough. Fold a towel and place it under your knees for more comfort and have a pillow close by for this exercise. If your bathroom is cramped, save this exercise for the living room floor.

GOOD FOR

Strengthening the spine, adductors, lats, quads, and hip flexors; activating the core, shoulder, and SI joint stabilizer muscles; improving stamina

VARIATION

Alternate lifting and lowering one foot at a time while your knees hover above the ground. Keep your hips stabilized to prevent them from tilting left or right.

1 Find the on-hands-and-knees position with proper body alignment. Pull your navel to the spine to activate your core, and direct your gaze toward the ground.

2 Place the pillow between your thighs, then tuck your toes under and squeeze the pillow between your legs. Lift both knees off the floor slightly so they hover above the ground.

3 Hold the position for 1 full inhale-exhale breath (see page 24). Then lower your knees back to the floor.

4 Repeat, completing 5 to 10 reps.

STANDING
QUAD STRETCH

Whether you run, bike, or sit all day at a desk, your quad muscles may be stiff and shortened. This stretch will lengthen your quads, and also improve knee flexibility. If you are not too steady on your feet, you can do the same stretch lying on your side.

GOOD FOR

Stretching the quads; improving knee flexibility

VARIATION

Once you are holding your foot, tuck your tailbone forward to feel a deeper stretch in the front upper thigh and hip flexor.

1 Stand tall facing the sink with your feet hip distance apart and your toes pointed forward; hold the sink with one hand for balance. Pull your navel to your spine to activate your core.

2 Lift your leg behind you, bending at the knee. Reach your arm on the same side behind you to grasp your foot in your hand. Activate your core to avoid arching your back.

3 Hold this position for 30 to 60 seconds. Gently release your foot to the ground.

4 Repeat on the other side.

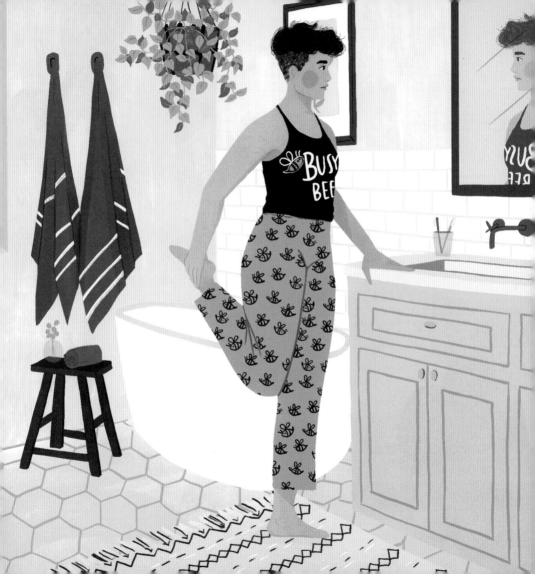

IN THE

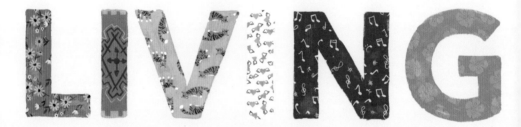

LIVING

So much living room furniture to use, so little time! All the floor exercises can be done on a mat, on a rug, or directly on the floor. You will need a sturdy chair, sofa, or coffee table; a pillow; and a soup can or light weight.

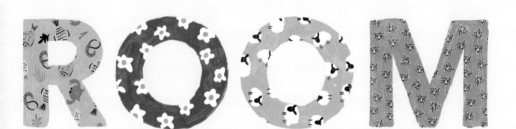

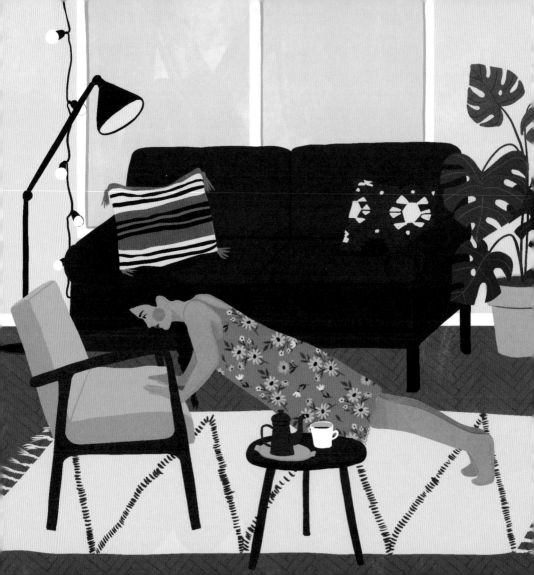

RBG'S DAILY PUSH-UP

A push-up is an exercise that strengthens your whole body. And, if the late Supreme Court Justice Ruth Bader Ginsburg could do these into her eighties, chances are you can too. You can modify this position by lowering your knees to the ground. You be the judge!

Strengthening the triceps, chest muscles, glutes, and quads; activating the core and shoulder stabilizer muscles; improving posture and stamina

Once you lower your body toward the sofa, add up and down pulses to your bent arms.

1 Kneel 3 to 4 steps away from your sofa or steady chair. Lean forward so that your hands are shoulder distance apart on the edge of the steady surface.

2 Open your chest and drop your shoulders away from your ears to feel an activation in the back of your shoulders and arms.

3 Tuck your toes and lift your knees off the floor into a plank position; actively engage your core.

4 Bend your elbows about 90 degrees to lower your body toward the sofa or chair, keeping your elbows pointed back. Then straighten your arms to return to the plank position.

5 Repeat, completing 10 to 12 reps.

SEATED ROLL BACK

This is a challenging abdominal exercise you can do sitting at your desk, passing time on a long flight, or watching TV late at night!

GOOD FOR

Strengthening the core, shoulder, spine stabilizer muscles, hip flexors, and obliques

VARIATIONS

Bring your arms forward or overhead.

Lift your feet off the floor, holding the backs of your thighs for support.

1 Sit at the edge of a chair with your upper body aligned and your feet flat on the floor. Press your feet into the ground.

2 Place your hands on the seat behind you, with your elbows slightly bent, fingers pointed forward, and shoulders away from your ears.

3 Pull your navel to the spine and shift your weight to the back of your sit bones, making room for an imaginary bowl of water to sit on your belly. Roll halfway down toward the chairback. As you roll, your spine will form a *J* shape.

4 Hold this position for 1 breath. Return to the starting position.

5 Repeat, completing 10 to 15 reps.

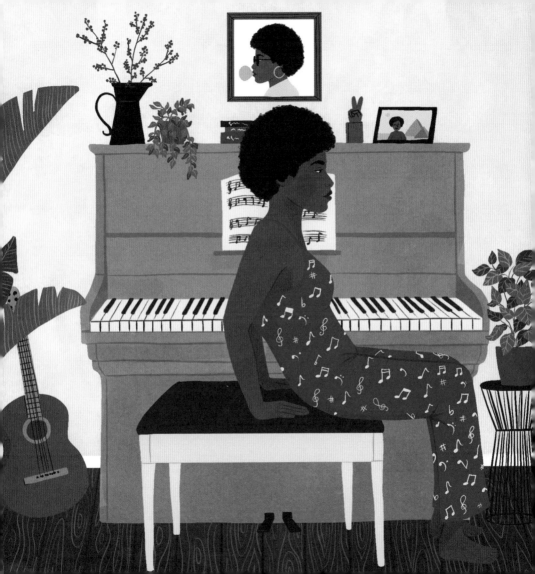

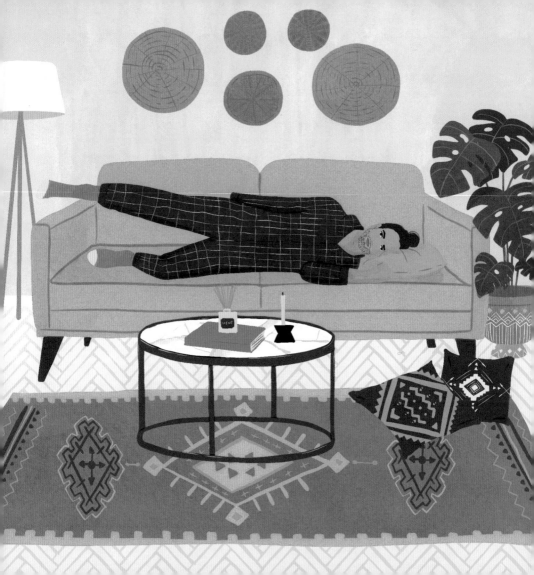

SIDE-LYING LEG LIFT

Side-lying exercises are essential for toning, strengthening, and aligning the hip and the knee. This exercise isolates and focuses on the hip muscles. Keep a pillow handy.

GOOD FOR

Strengthening the hip abductors and glutes; activating the core and hip stabilizer muscles; improving balance

VARIATIONS

Place your top hand against your thigh, providing resistance for your leg to push against as it lifts.

Extend your bottom leg to challenge your alignment and balance.

1 Lie on your side with proper body alignment on a rug, mat, or sofa, supporting your head with a pillow. Bend your bottom arm and rest it on the floor or under the pillow for extra head support. Bend your bottom leg and place your top arm on your side.

2 Lift and lower your top leg while keeping your bottom leg on the floor.

3 Repeat, completing 10 reps, then switch, completing 10 reps on the other side.

SIDE-LYING BEND AND EXTEND

Get into the action with the Side-Lying Bend and Extend! You can do this on a rug or mat or, if you want to be really comfy, on the sofa. Keep a pillow handy.

GOOD FOR

Activating the core; strengthening the abductors and glutes; increasing hip mobility; stabilizing the hip and spine; improving balance

VARIATION

Extend your bottom leg; this will challenge your alignment and balance.

1 Lie on your side with proper body alignment, supporting your head with a pillow. Bend your bottom arm and rest it on the floor or under the pillow for extra head support. Bend your bottom leg and place your top arm on your side.

2 Lift your top leg to hip level, keeping it straight and parallel to the ground. Then bend it at the knee and hip joints to create 90-degree angles.

3 Straighten and extend your lifted upper leg while maintaining hip, knee, and foot alignment.

4 Repeat, completing 10 reps, then switch, completing 10 reps on the other side.

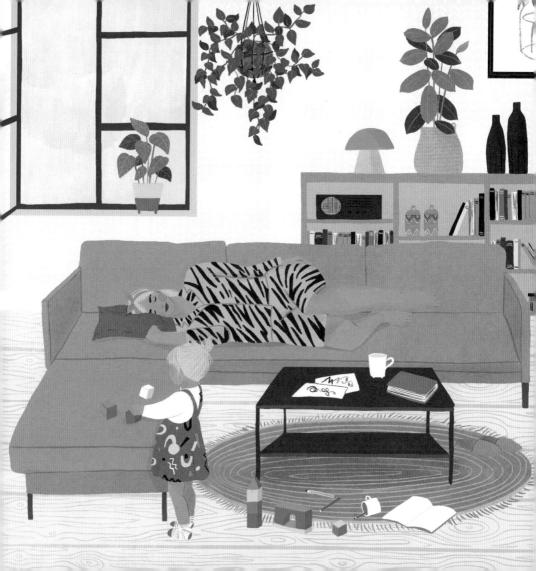

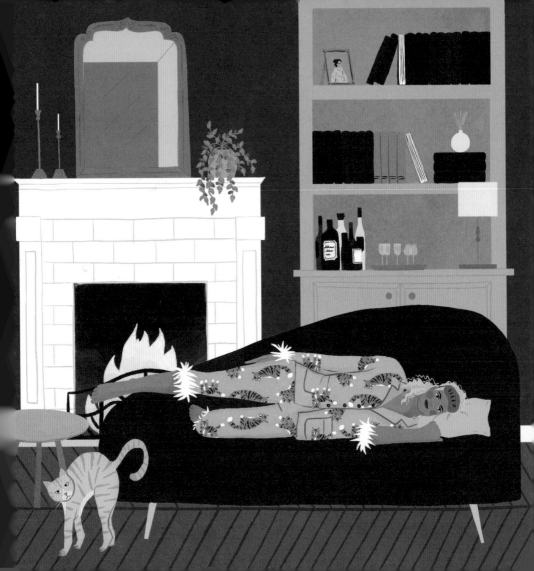

SIDE-LYING LEG CIRCLE

Your hip muscles may be a little fatigued after the previous side-lying exercises, but you will experience benefits from exploring the movement of your thigh bone in your hip joint. You can massage your hip muscles after this exercise to help them recover.

GOOD FOR

Activating the core; strengthening the abductors and glutes; increasing hip mobility; stabilizing the hip and spine; improving balance

VARIATION

Extend your bottom leg; this will challenge your alignment and balance.

1 Lie on your side with proper body alignment, supporting your head with a pillow. Bend your bottom arm and rest it on the floor or under the pillow for extra head support. Bend your bottom leg and place your top arm on your side.

2 Bend both knees at about 45 degrees, keeping your legs together.

3 Straighten and raise your top leg, keeping your foot at hip level. Then make a small circle, moving your leg from the hip joint.

4 Repeat, completing 5 reps clockwise and 5 reps counterclockwise, then switch, completing 5 reps clockwise and 5 reps counterclockwise on the other side.

NOT·A·CROWD·PLEASER TEASER

This exercise is typically called The Teaser, but one of my clients jokingly renamed it the "Not-a-Crowd-Pleaser Teaser"! Try saying that 5 times fast. If this exercise is challenging for you, consider starting slowly; it will eventually become doable.

GOOD FOR

Strengthening the hip flexors, core muscles, quads, and calves; activating the shoulder and spine stabilizer muscles

VARIATIONS

Fully extend your legs straight and keep them together with pointed toes.

Bring your arms forward or overhead while you do the exercise.

1 Sit on the edge of the sofa with your hands resting on the edge and your fingers pointed forward.

2 Activate your core by bringing your navel to your spine. Tuck your tailbone to shift your weight to the back of your sit bones.

3 Lift your legs one at a time with bent knees. Reach your arms forward, with your chest open and your shoulders wide. For extra support, hold the backs of your thighs.

4 Remain in this position for 3 breaths and then lower your legs one at a time to the starting position.

5 Repeat, completing 3 to 5 reps.

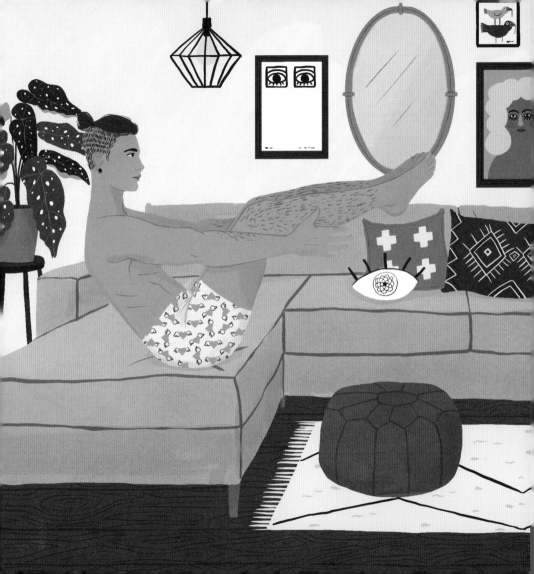

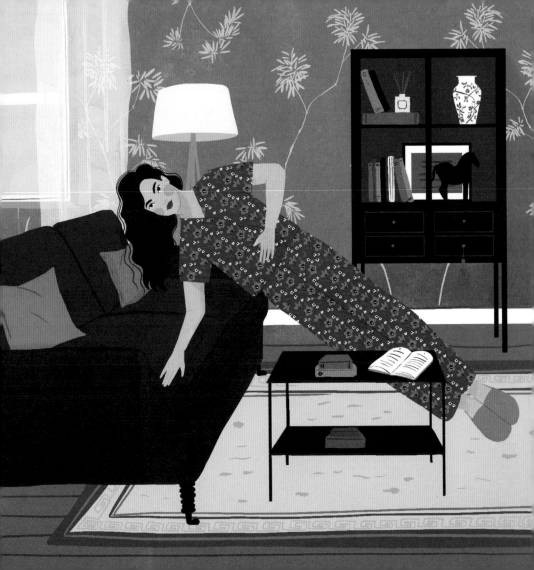

SOFA SIDE PLANK

What's more challenging than Standing Plank (page 49)? Sofa Side Plank! In this plank exercise, the challenge is to balance on one side of your body with your only support coming from your forearm on the sofa and your feet on the floor. It will strengthen your core more than any other exercise. Keep a soup can handy for the variation.

GOOD FOR

Strengthening the glutes, abductors, adductors, obliques, and triceps; activating the core, spine, and shoulder stabilizer muscles

VARIATION

Lift and lower your upper arm and leg. For an extra challenge, hold a soup can in your upper hand. Complete 10 reps.

1 Kneel sideways half a step away from the sofa. Place your forearm closest to the sofa on the edge with your palm facing down, and your elbow directly below your shoulder.

2 Without moving, *think* about drawing your lower elbow toward your rib cage to stabilize the shoulder joint.

3 Extend the leg farthest from the sofa and then the other leg so that both legs and feet are stacked together. Activate your core to balance on your forearm and feet. Hold this position for 10 to 30 seconds.

4 Repeat on the other side.

SWAN DIVE PREP

Swan Dive Prep, a warm-up for the classic Pilates exercise of the same name, opens your chest and stretches your abdominals. Activate your core and keep your abdominals engaged throughout the movement to help protect your back. Keep a pillow handy for the variation.

GOOD FOR

Strengthening the spine extensors, core, glutes, pectoral muscles, triceps, and biceps; activating the spine and shoulder stabilizer muscles

VARIATION

As you bend your arms and lower your upper torso toward the floor, you can lift one leg at a time upward. Then try to lift both legs. If needed, place a pillow under your hips for comfort.

1 Lie on your stomach with your forehead resting on your mat, your palms facing down just below shoulder level, and your elbows bent, pointing out and back.

2 Rotate your legs out and wider than hip distance apart. Point your toes to activate your legs.

3 Activate your core and push on the mat with both hands to straighten your arms and begin to lift your upper body off the ground. Depending on your flexibility, your head, chest, and rib cage may lift.

4 After lifting your upper body to your comfort level, return to the starting position.

5 Repeat, completing 5 to 10 reps.

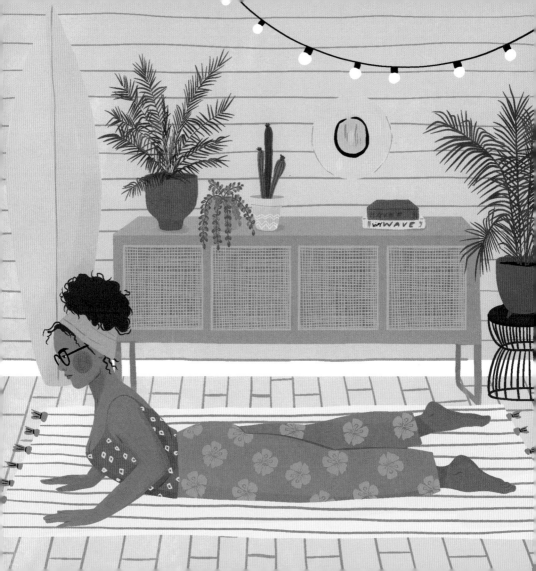

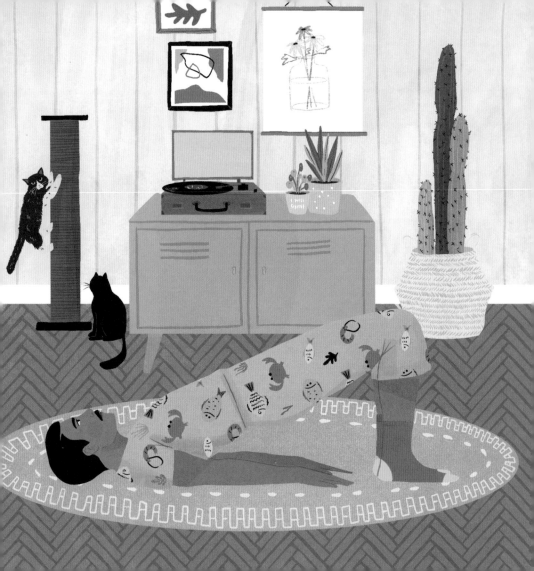

"GLUTE"-CAMP BRIDGE

This exercise is like a mini boot camp for your glutes. Glutes play a key role in proper walking, standing, and sitting, and are the propulsive force behind running. Strong glutes support your lower back in many different movements and prevent injuries. Power to the glutes; they have your back!

GOOD FOR

Strengthening the glutes and hamstrings; activating the core, spine, and shoulder stabilizer muscles

VARIATION

While your spine is raised, lift one leg to tabletop, keeping your hips level, and hold for a breath, then lower the leg. Switch and repeat with the other leg. That is 1 rep. Repeat, completing 3 to 5 reps.

1 Lie down on your back with proper body alignment, palms facing in or down, whichever is more comfortable. Place your feet flat on the mat, with your knees bent, and your legs parallel and hip distance apart.

2 Press your feet into the mat to activate your hamstrings and glutes, and lift your back off the mat. Align your knees with your hips, ribs, and chest, while keeping your head, shoulders, and arms on the mat for stability.

3 Hold this position for 1 breath and feel an activation in your glutes. Return to the starting position.

4 Repeat, completing 10 to 15 reps.

ABDOMINALS CHALLENGE

Pace yourself for this exercise and its even more difficult variations. I promise your core will smile at the end! You'll need a pillow for this exercise.

GOOD FOR

Strengthening the adductors, abductors, quads, hip flexors, and obliques; activating the core, spine, and shoulder stabilizer muscles

VARIATIONS

From step 2, lift one leg toward your chest while lowering the other toward the floor, then switch. Repeat, completing 10 to 15 reps.

From step 2, circle both your legs away from each other once. Repeat, completing 10 to 15 reps, then switch, completing 10 to 15 reps in the opposite direction.

1 Lie down on your back with proper body alignment and palms facing down. Place a pillow under your hips to support your sacrum and lumbar spine, and provide extra comfort.

2 Pull your navel to your spine and imprint your lumbar spine. Lift one leg at a time to tabletop position and then straighten both legs.

3 Lower your legs to either side, away from your midline, only so far that your lumbar spine stays imprinted. Then slowly bring them back together.

4 Repeat, completing 10 reps.

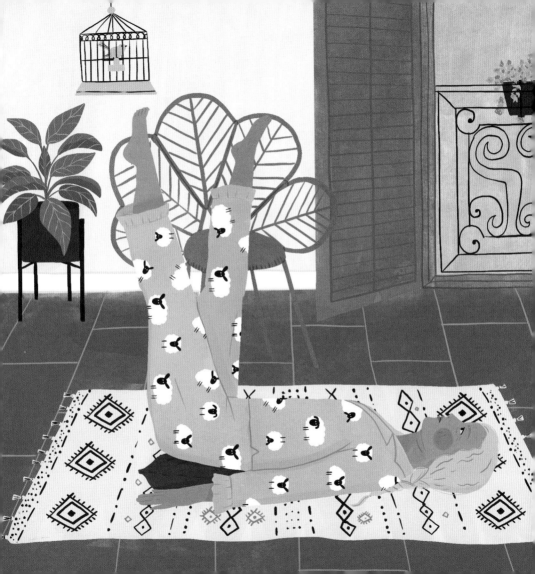

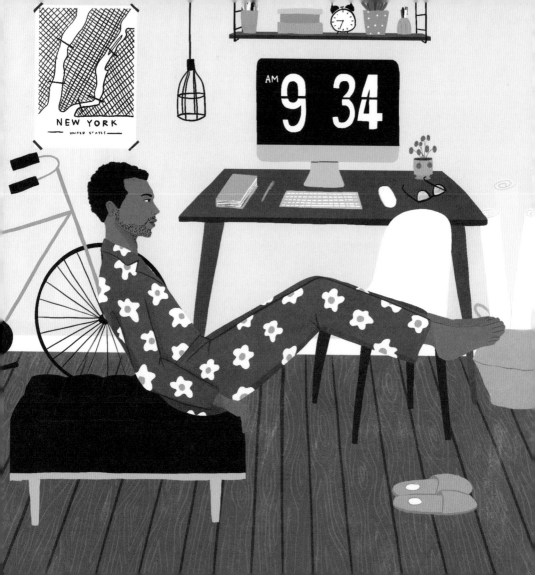

HIP CIRCLE

This is a sneaky exercise that is more than just circling your hips. It may even feel like you're not circling them at all but only rotating your knees. Don't let that fool you! You are really strengthening your core and hip stabilizers and lubricating your joints.

GOOD FOR

Strengthening the core, triceps, lats, obliques, adductors, abductors, quads, and hip flexors

VARIATIONS

Make bigger circles, maintaining a stabilized pelvis.

Make circles with straightened legs for an even greater challenge.

1 Sit on the edge of the sofa with hands gripping the edge and arms slightly bent at the elbows.

2 Pull your navel to the spine and tuck your tailbone forward, shifting your weight to the back of your sit bones.

3 Lift one leg and then lift the other to join the first, balancing on your sit bones and keeping your knees slightly bent just below shoulder level. Open your chest and drop your shoulders away from your ears.

4 Moving from the hips, draw small circles with your legs together in a clockwise motion.

5 Repeat, completing 5 to 10 reps, then switch, completing 5 to 10 reps going counterclockwise.

COFFEE TABLE SIDE KICK

This kick is not quite a martial-arts move, but is definitely a useful exercise for anyone who wants to strengthen their obliques and glutes. Place a pillow under your forearm for extra comfort.

GOOD FOR

Strengthening the obliques, lats, hip flexors, and glutes; activating the core, spine, shoulder, hip, and sacroiliac joint stabilizer muscles

VARIATIONS

Add up and down pulses to the extended leg, keeping your heel aligned with your knee and hip.

Bend your extended leg 90 degrees at the hip and knee, then straighten it back to the starting position.

1 Start by kneeling sideways a half step away from the coffee table (or sofa).

2 Place the forearm closest to the table down on the edge, with your palm facing down and your elbow directly below your shoulder.

3 Extend your outside leg away from the table and lift it off the floor. Distribute your weight between your forearm and the knee that remains on the floor.

4 Kick your lifted leg forward, from the hip, and then bring it back behind your upper body and torso, while stabilizing your spine and pelvis.

5 Repeat, completing 10 to 15 reps, then switch, completing 10 to 15 reps on the other side.

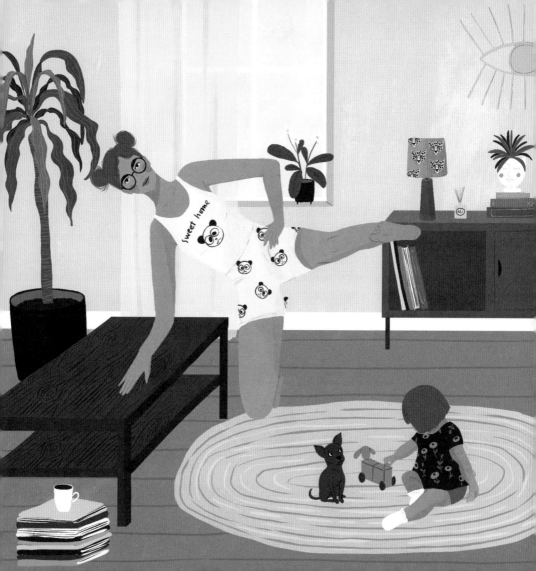

ROUTINES

Many of my clients come to me with common aches and pains from years of overuse or strains from repetitive action. I've designed a handful of specialized routines for these common conditions using exercises found throughout the book. I hope you find a favorite routine here; if not, make up your own using the "Good for" sections throughout the book as a guide! I recommend using the bedroom workout as a warm-up and modifying the routine to fit your environment and comfort.

FOR DESK SITTERS

Sitting for long periods of time can lead to tight hip flexors, weak glutes, a sore lower back, and eventually injuries. Minimize the time you sit, use a good ergonomic chair, and practice these simple exercises on your break.

FOR BACK PAIN

The spine needs to be stable and flexible at the same time. Sitting, bad posture, repetitive movements, and lack of core strength can cause imbalances and back pain. Whether you lift heavy bags of dirt, move boxes, or just have a sensitive back, your spine will love this series of exercises!

FOR ATHLETES

If you run a marathon, swim laps at the pool, hike a steep mountain, or golf on weekends, this routine is for you! You will feel empowered, aligned, energized, and ready for any high-intensity activity.

FOR GARDENERS

Gardening is exercise! You move in all directions—pulling weeds, lifting heavy pots, and holding awkward positions. You need training for that just like you would when preparing for a game, race, or swim. Here are some exercises that may help you get down into the *weeds*.

FOR BALANCE

As a circus performer, I used to practice how to fall, and now I do the opposite—I teach people how to prevent falls. Here are exercises that will help you improve balance, core strength, and steadiness on your feet.

FOR FLEXIBILITY

When we talk about flexibility—the ability to move the body in all directions with ease—we also talk about fascia, the soft connective tissue that holds your body together. With injuries, aging, or lack of movement, your fascia can become stuck, resulting in poor body mechanics and possibly pain. These exercises allow you to stretch and roll out the fascia.

FOR PREGNANCY

When expecting, it is essential to focus on alignment, organic movement, and strengthening your core to support your back. These exercises boost your energy, improve your posture, and help you carry with ease. Please avoid exercises that require lying on your stomach over the whole gestation period and lying on your back in the second and third trimester.

(In the second and third trimester, you can do this sitting on a chair or an exercise ball.)

FOR NEW MOMS

After 6 to 12 weeks of having your little bundle of joy, it may be time to gently rebuild your core. Listen to your body: You may need more or less time to recover. At any rate, performing the inhale-exhale breathing exercise allows your body to center and heal faster.

ACKNOWLEDGMENTS

I would like to thank all my fantastic friends and clients at Begin Pilates for their support and dedication. Very special thanks to Kacie Dart and Susan Hodge for being my always available sounding boards and to Carly Larsson for helping me shape the early stages of this book with such enthusiasm; also to Janell, Monika, Paula, Sandra, and Ruth for always being there. A big cheer to the amazing Chronicle Books team, especially Rachel Hiles and Maddy Wong. Gratitude to my lovely daughters, Alina and Imogene, and my wonderful husband, Danny, for their love and encouragement.